How I Ran My First Marathon

By Yolanda Hill

Copyright © 2014 by Yolanda Hill

YOLANDA HILL PUBLICATIONS

Cover Design by: Tamika Hall

ISBN-10: 1499561407

ISBN-13: 978-1499561401

DEDICATION

This book is dedicated to My Lord and Savior Jesus Christ who lives on the inside of me. He put running in my feet to run the race. The Bible says in Hebrews 12:1, "Therefore we also, since we are surrounded by so great a cloud of witnesses, let us lay aside every weight, and the sin which so easily ensnares us, and let us run with endurance the race that is set before us," Also, a special thank you to my mother, Nina Hill, my friends Lorre Meek and Jannelle Dennison for their awesome support on my first marathon day!

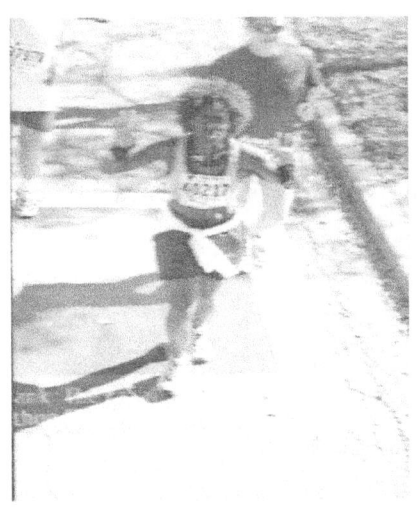

To those who have never walked or run before but would like to do so, this is the book for you.

Go to the link below to receive 5 marathon tips

http://forms.aweber.com/form/39/207 6793339.htm

TABLE OF CONTENTS

CHAPTER ONE:

GETTING STARTED

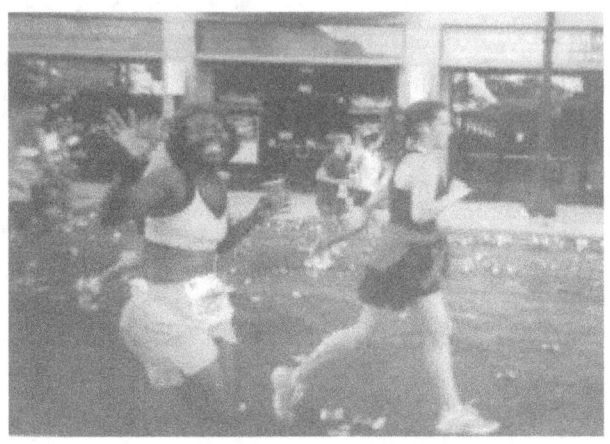

I have always been the type of person who believes in getting some form of exercise. Why? Well, it's good for the body and mind. I have worked out at the health club for exercise for years. One day, I thought, it would be nice to add something different to my exercise routine, other than biking on stationary bikes, toning on machines and participating in cardio classes.

When I walked on treadmills at the health club, I discovered that walking outdoors is much different.

There is a large track near my home, so I began to walk around it for so many laps that would equal to a mile or more. I discovered that there were other people that enjoyed walking around the track, early in the morning. This was good, because I didn't have to worry about being alone while exercising at this time of morning.

Early morning walking is good to start off your day. In the summer months, early morning is better because it's very uncomfortable to walk in the heat and it can be unsafe. Many people also choose to walk in the evenings, because it is cooler at that time of day.

At work, I was asked by my superior, to represent my unit with a fundraiser. The event was the March of Dimes–Walk America. Initially, I was hesitant because I knew this project would involve some work. Once I thought the idea through, I realized it would be a well-invested project for the following reasons:

1. It was a good cause.
2. It would be a challenge. The project would cause me to come out of my comfort zone and ask people to support an event that would benefit someone less fortunate than themselves.
3. I would have the opportunity to make a difference in someone else's life.

4. I would get some good exercise, as well.

Fundraising

Participating in a marathon carries an expense. This is not an expense you have to carry alone. Many runners will acquire sponsors. The same applies for charity walks. Asking for support wasn't as difficult as I thought. These are the steps I used to raise funds for this event:

1. I let the potential sponsors know what I was doing and why. For example, "I am a walker for the March of Dimes-Walk America! Will you make a donation today to help children who are born with birth defects?"

2. Decide how much support you need to raise?

3. Once the people commit to supporting the walk, give a special show of recognition for support by posting a special-designed paper shoe with their name indicated on it and post on a window or board of an office to show number of supporters.

4. Complete fundraising support by the specified date.

5. Be determined to walk and finish. Don't let your sponsors' donations be made in vain.

Preparing for the walk:

- Get up early and stretch
- Glass of orange juice, oatmeal and bagel with jelly.

- Dress for the walk: (T-shirts were provided for walkers), sweat pants or shorts, socks and walking shoes, sun visor or hat, sunglasses for sun glare.

The day of my first walk event was exciting because there were so many people involved: families, babies in strollers, kids, teens, and adults younger and older. Pets were also included in this event – dogs on leashes! It was amazing to see the numbers that supported this event! Once the walk began, it was great because you got to view scenic parts of the city as you talked and walked with other participants.

At the end of the three to six mile walk, I was quite tired but I was excited to have finished. A volunteer for March of Dimes congratulated me for finishing and I received a finisher's tag.

Once I returned to work the next day, I let the supporters know that I completed the walk and I shared the event details that took place following the walk. I also sent out a letter of appreciation for their monetary support that helped babies that were born with birth defects.

Since I successfully completed that event, I was asked to represent my assigned unit by raising support and participating in other events scheduled for the calendar year such as: Special Olympics Torch Run, The Run to Remember, and The UNCF Walk-, Run-, Skate or Bike-a-thon.

For many years, I have supported and participated in many of the charity walks and runs and I still support them from time to time.

CHAPTER TWO:

JOINING A TRAINING PROGRAM

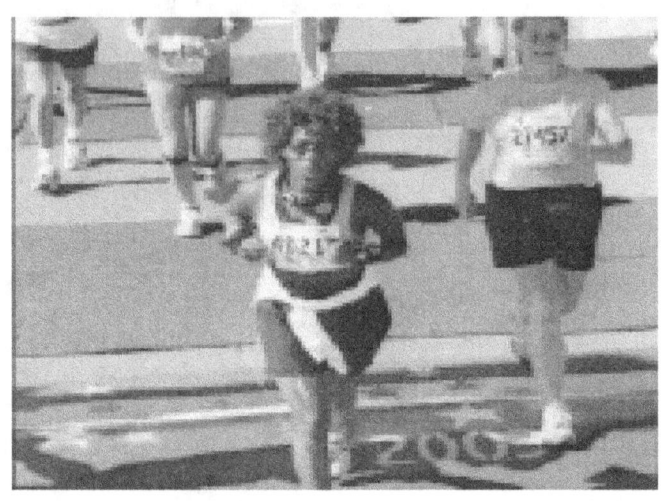

It came to a point when I felt like it was time to move on to something a little more challenging. I always wondered if I could do a distance run. I decided I wanted to take on a challenge of walking or running a distance race of between five to ten miles. This is something I had never done but wished I could, so I decided to join a running group. I went through many groups before finding one that fit my needs.

The first group that I tried to join turned me down saying I didn't qualify because I didn't have enough running experience. They suggested that I apply the following year and join their beginner's running program.

I wasn't quite satisfied with that answer; so, I began to seek out other running groups. I was referred to a running group that seemed to be what I needed at the time. The name of the group was Chicago Endurance Sport (CES).

I decided to go with this group because I liked their presentation, their orientation for new members, and what they offered as a running group. What was so exciting and encouraging to me about this training group was that they worked with a person at the level that one was at.

I registered for the 12-week training program to prepare for The Chicago Distance Classic Race. The program included coaches to help one find the running or run/walk training right for them and they guided them through the training process step by step.

The CES training program included two coached workouts for endurance, focusing on improving running form and speed.

The one thing I appreciated about CES is that water and Gatorade was provided at all these hydration stations at every three to five-mile mark.

Usually there was someone standing near the table to hand you your drink while you ran/walked by. There were energy bars (Clif Bars) and gel shots (small packets of carbs to be taken with water for energy), as well.

As the weeks went by, thank the Lord, I began to see improvement in my running and keeping up with the group at the pace that we started off with, a 14-mile pace. The pace time is the amount of time (minutes/seconds) it takes a runner to complete 1 mile.

The Tuesday/weekday practices concentrated on speedwork and strengthening. Speedwork is any running workout in which you run faster than your normal pace for a certain time or distance also called intervals. In between those fast intervals, you typically recover at a slower than normal pace. ("Speedwork" by Christine Luff www.about.com) At times this was challenging for me, because I would train after working an eight-hour day. The long runs were always done on Sunday mornings. For me, this was not convenient because I enjoyed attending church on Sunday; therefore, I became even more motivated to run a lot faster so that I could at least get to hear some of the message before the end of the morning service at church.

In time, (within 6-8 weeks) I began to notice that my pace improved and I was able to run at a faster pace than some of the people in my group. Once I realized my progress in the beginner's group, I decided it was time to move on to the intermediate level.

I joined the intermediate level group, met the group leader, and decided to try to keep up with her pace. It was a little bit challenging at first to keep up with the new group's pace, but in time, I was even able to keep up with the leader.

During the practice runs, people often conversed about various races that they had participated in. I loved this time, because I was able to find out the scoop on what was happening with upcoming races and events. Most of the time I enjoyed just listening because

I tire more quickly while talking and I really needed every bit of energy I had.

I was surprised to learn that, when the weather is not so favorable, a scheduled practice or race may not be cancelled. The group laughed at me and told me that cancellations don't happen too often. One day the opportunity presented itself, I had to run in the rain and it was very uncomfortable for me. It was hard for me to focus in conditions like that. Nonetheless, I survived and finished the run. II Timothy 2:5, "An also if anyone competes in athletics, he is not crowned unless he competes according to the rules."

In addition to the scheduled easy stretch and run days; Monday, Wednesday and Friday of each week, I also did speedwork with my running group on Tuesdays. On Thursday's I cross-trained at the health club. I enjoyed aerobic classes and utilizing the weight machines to help strengthen muscle tone in my arms and legs. Additionally, I enjoyed biking workouts on the track near my home. By the end of the 12-week training period, I felt confident that I would be able to complete this race.

While preparing for the Chicago Distance Classic Race, I was assigned to the Beginner's Run/Walk group for training. The people I met were nice. Most of the runners that were assigned to this group were training for the first time, like me, and one or two others had trained at this level before. One day a week, (Tuesdays) I meet with my group to prepare for our weekday speed work practice. The group started off walking for a very short distance, and then we began to increase our speed and runs for longer distances. These speed runs were repeated a number of times during the practice. Our time was tracked by the alarm on our watches, which were designed specifically for this kind of practice run.

While running with my group, I noticed that I was the slowest one in the group especially for one of the practice runs when we concentrated on hill work. That was very challenging for me, to the point that I felt like running off to the side of one of the hills to rest a bit. But instead, I resisted that temptation and pressed my way to finish the run. Now my body began to feel like I was going to have an asthma attack. I found myself thinking, "Wow, this is tiring, to run without stopping "are we there yet? Is it time to walk yet?" Needless to say, I barely finished that practice.

The following Sunday, I met up with my group bright and early at 7:30 A.M. for the assigned long run day. The group leader explained the route we were to take and when we needed to complete the run. I started out ok. At least I was able to keep up with the group for a while. Then I began to feel real heavy. My legs felt especially heavy and it seemed that I couldn't pick up any speed. I found out, later, that my form for running was incorrect and that I should be applying the heel-toe method of running because it gives the runner more speed. Unfortunately, at this point, I hadn't attended any of the running clinics yet. I didn't feel like I could make it to the finish line. A group of runners, along the course, stopped to make sure I was ok. I felt embarrassed that I seemed to be the only one struggling to complete my first practice long run. Then, one particular young lady decided to run with me to the finish line. God bless her. She asked me what I had eaten three days prior to the race and the day before. I explained that I didn't hydrate much, I had soda pop and I had eaten ribs, potato salad, hot links, baked beans and desert the day prior to this long run. She explained to me those foods were not good to eat the day before a race, especially a long run. Instead, she said that I should have started hydrating and preparing my body with carbohydrates (vegetables, fruits, whole grains, fiber and protein) at least three days prior to the run and especially the day before the race. If you are thinking about running any distance run, I would highly recommend joining a training program. When looking for a program, look for one that includes:

- Daily training schedule and log
- Nutrition log to help you reach your desired goal
- Explanation of training peaks
- Experienced coaches
- Personalized training schedules

CHAPTER THREE:

CLINICS & SEMINARS

Clinics and seminars will help you safely reach your goals and give you instruction on a variety of topics:

- Good Form Running - become a faster, more efficient runner
- Benefits of Yoga for Runners
- Tools And Gadgets For Endurance Runners (GPS Heart Rate monitors)
- Tricks For Speedy Long Run Recovery
- Core And Strength Training
- Injury Prevention And Flexibility
- Food As Fuel: Sports Nutrition
- Mental Skills Training
- Comprehensive Race Prep

These clinics were very informative regarding:

- **Shoes-** I discovered that I wore shoes too small for many years. I learned that the shoes I wore should have been a half size larger. The reason for this is, when you run, especially for a long distance, your feet swell.

- **Special Socks-** I also learned that I needed to wear special double layered socks for running to help eliminate blisters on my feet. Blisters were always a problem for me while running. I used blister pads on areas prone to blisters.

- **Running Form-** When I ran, my form was improper in that I was a flat-footed runner. I learned that was part of the reason I had difficulty picking up speed.

One way to identify if a person is running improperly is when you can clearly hear the individual running. The correct form I used for running was the heel-toe method, as it gives more speed.

I also learned that proper form and posture requires a runner to run holding their head upward for plenty of oxygen (air). When a person runs with their head down, like hump back, they are not getting enough air in their lungs for good running. In addition to that, one must swing their arms back and forth for speed, never side to side, because this method will slow one down. Chin up, pump the arms and one can make it to the finish line!

- **Clothing** - I learned that I needed to change my attire. What I wore for running was cute, and well coordinated, but not proper for running. I experienced chafing (peeling away of skin) on various parts of my body as a result. The runner's apparel should be synthetic, lightweight, breathable clothing that wicks moisture away from your skin. It is great to be able to complete a run without the chafing. A Sun visor/hat worn with sunglasses is always good to keep sun out of your face. Be sure to wear sun block to protect your skin as well.

- **Body Glide -** This product is great to help eliminate chafing, while you run. It is a type of hard gel that you rub on the areas of your body prone to chafing quickly.

- **Gel shots -** good for long runs. They are small tubes of carb gel or chews taken orally with water every five miles or more.   It gives you that energy you need to keep running.

- **Fanny packs -** should be worn during runs for storing your necessities while running.

- **Running Computer or GPS –** is a special watch (I used the Polar RS200 brand) worn by runners to help track their pace, time, speed, calories, special timer alarm, heart rate, etc. It is a very helpful tool to use when running. This device help runners to better concentrate on their race.

- **Stretching** - before and after the run is very important. This also helps prevent injury while running. If you do not, you will probably experience tight and sore muscles which will slow you down and prevent you from performing your best when you need to do your weekly workouts, speed-work, and long runs. I learned this the hard way. Unfortunately, the very first week of my training, I experienced tight and sore muscles because I didn't stretch properly. It takes a little time to recuperate from this type of injury. Your time is valuable and should be used very wisely when training for races. The last thing you need is a distraction that will slow you down.

- **Massages** – I learned that massages are good for runners. I will list 10 reason why:
  1. Dilates blood vessels which promotes circulation and lowers blood pressure
  2. Assists venous blood flow
  3. Promotes rapid removal of metabolic waste products
  4. Improves the oxygen carrying capacity of red blood cell
  5. Improves pulmonary function by loosening tight respiratory muscles

6. Reduces muscle soreness and fatigue
7. Increases/restores joint range of motion
8. Reduces cortisol levels and norepinephrine and epinephrine levels
9. Restores posture and gait
10. Improves connective tissues healing. (Susan Paul, <u>Runner's World</u> Magazine, Dec 27, 2013)

It was truly worth attending the clinics and workshops for runners. My approach to running was changed from that point forward. My new goal was to run injury free races each time.

CHAPTER FOUR:

DANGERS IN RUNNING

While the joy of running is great, if you are not prepared for it there are many dangers associated with the sport. Listed below are eight injuries that are common among runners:

- Stress fractures
- Shin splints
- Achilles tendinitis
- Muscle pull
- Heat exhaustion and hyperthermia (fever or extremely high body temperature)
- Ankle sprain
- Iliotibial Band Syndrome (ITBS) - an injury caused when the muscle that extends from the outside of

the pelvis to under the knee
becomes irritated

During my 18-week training for the Chicago Marathon, I did encounter some unpleasant experiences. I have always been prone to blisters. I used blisters pads and double layered socks to help eliminate this problem.

I also experienced hyperthermia during one of my summer morning races. It was very, very hot that morning and I thought that I hydrated enough, but soon I found out that I didn't. As I ran, I started feeling nauseated, dizzy, and weak. I almost fainted. I stopped and hydrated with water and especially Gatorade (to put electrolytes back into my body) in addition to wetting my head and body with water for some cool relief. After a while, I felt better, but it was one of the worst feelings I ever experienced.

CHAPTER FIVE:

THE RUNNER'S EXPO

Usually a day or two prior to the race, the runners are required to pick up their gear package at the "Runner's Expo." Upon arrival, each runner receives a bag that contains several items such as a t-shirt, bib number, Body Glide, gel shots, energy bars, timing chip, and advertisings for other races. A timing chip is an electronic device that allows the marathon coordinators to provide runners with the net time it takes to finish the race. It starts once the runners cross the starting line and stops once the runners cross the finish line.

Runners may also participate in a number of activities at the expo, such as having their pictures taken and watching videos of races from the prior year. It's always amazing to watch how some of the many elite runners (The Kenyans) and others, run with such excellent form, strength and stamina.

Normally, a large number of vendors are available at these expos to sell products like running shoes, socks, running apparel with the moisture-wicking features, gel shots, granola bars, sunglasses, Body Glide, sun visors, hats, Tylenol samples, various juices and nutritional foods. There are many restaurant stations available for attendees of the expo as well as seminars on how to prepare for your race before and after your run. Physical therapists (Athletico) and other vendors were available to demonstrate how to use various devices that will help prevent injuries prior to your run. I received some good information regarding the importance of massages and a complimentary massage as well.

The expo is also a good time to network with other groups and runners. There is so much to learn from everything available at the expo.

CHAPTER SIX:

CHICAGO DISTANCE CLASSIC

The day of the Chicago Distance Classic had arrived. I woke up early to thank God for another day and to get prepared for the race. I felt a little nervous on the inside. I kept reciting Philippians 4:13 to myself, *"I can do all things through Christ who strengthens me."* I started out with a good carbohydrate breakfast, (8 oz. glass of orange juice, a bagel, banana and 8 oz. yogurt, 2-3 hours prior to race) drank water and plenty of stretching. I checked to make sure I had all my gear and I applied Body Glide to areas where it was needed. I included my runners socks, blister pads (to prevent possible blistering), gym shoes with the timing chip laced between my shoe laces, the bib number pinned onto the front of my tank top, and a supply of gel shots to be used at certain water stations of the race.

I arrived early to the race location. I had never seen so many people, young and old. I desperately searched for my running group, but with no success. There were so many runners participating in this race that it was difficult to find anyone.

I started the race without my group. I didn't begin my race too fast because it is wise to save some energy for the end. I implemented the things I learned about form and pace. I began the heel-toe method while running and was still looking out for my running group. During this time, I recall seeing a tall, dark and lean young man, running alone on the other side of the running course. I thought, "Wow, he must be lost. Why is he on that side of the course?" I was later informed, at the end of race that the young man I thought was lost, was an elite runner from Kenya and he was on the other side of the course already because he was that far ahead of everyone else.

At about the 6-mile mark, I finally spotted my group on the other side of the course. I waved and they were surprised to see me alone on the other side of course.

While running, I keep my mind occupied and thinking of other runners who may need more strength to finish the race. I offered up special, short prayers. I learned to encourage myself with the following key scriptures from the Holy Bible:

- Colossians 3:23-24 -"Whatever you do, work heartily, as for the Lord and not for men, knowing that from the Lord you will receive the inheritance as your reward you are serving the Lord Christ."
- Romans 8:37 – "Nay, *in all these things we are more than conquerors through Him that loved us.*"
- II Timothy 4:7 – "*I have fought the good fight, I have finished the race, I have kept the faith.*"

Finally, I can see the finish line. Hallelujah! I crossed the finish line and received my medal for completing my first long run of 12 miles. I felt a real sense of accomplishment.

After completing The Chicago Distance Classic, I was ready for another level in running. I decided that I would like to run the Chicago Marathon which is 26.2 miles.

CHAPTER SEVEN:

THE MARATHON EXPERIENCE

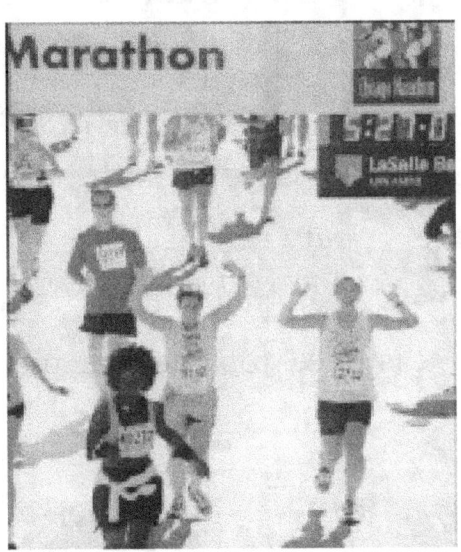

I registered for the Chicago Marathon right away. I did this for a few reasons. First, after finishing the Chicago Distance Classic, I felt like I could accomplish anything. Secondly, registration for this popular race fills up quickly.

I knew that once I completed the training program, I was ready for the marathon. The training for the marathon was a lot similar to the training I went through for the Chicago Distance Classic Race (12 mile run). The difference between the training programs is that the training is longer and the distance for the practice runs are longer and more intense.

I want to give you an idea of what my first marathon was like to help you, as much as possible, be fully prepared for yours. When I made the decision to register for this race I also registered with CES for another training program, this time it was an 18-week training program for the Marathon. I felt very confident that their training program would help me better prepare and complete my 26.2-mile race.

As I was training for the Marathon, I realized that I was ready for another pair of running shoes. Shoes are needed after every 300 miles. In order to get the best performance out of one's running shoes, it is advisable for a runner to replace them this often, because it will help them to run their best, while training.

A personal training log is good to use to keep record of your progress while training for a marathon. A finishing time goal is important. What helped me decide on a finishing time was the following: I was informed that if a runner does not complete the marathon within a designated time frame, the barricades that clear the path in the streets will open for traffic and the runner's name and time for completing the race will not be indicated in the newspaper. On that note, I decide my goal for completing my race will be 5 hours.

I recall an incident that occurred at one of my races. Caution: Never wear something new on the day of a race that you have not worn during your practice run. Needless to say, I wore a pair of new, but cute running shorts on the day of the race. The short's kept ridding up my legs and I had to keep pulling them down. After a while, I felt myself getting chaff and there was no body glide available! "Oh no!" So I started trying to run wide-legged, which was awkward. The next thing I know, I tripped, and began to roll down the running path. Fortunately, no one tripped over me. Note: periodically check your shoes for possible loose or untied laces during the course of your run. I found out the hard way. Once I stopped rolling, I was a little dusty of course; I found out that my fall was caused by an untied shoelace. I quickly tied my lace and tried to find my pace group. A pace group is identified by the lead pacer of the group holding a sign with the group's pace time on it. The pace time is the amount of time (minutes/seconds) it takes a runner to complete 1 mile. Unfortunately, they were nowhere within view.

Sometimes, unfortunately circumstances just happen, it comes with the sport of running. The goal is to run smart and safe by applying what is learned in your training clinics.

The day of the big race was finally here! I was actually going to run my first Chicago Marathon! The morning started off with prayer, a good carb breakfast two hours prior to the race, (orange juice, bagel, eggs, oatmeal, banana and water) and much stretching. I made sure that I had everything that I needed: My tank top, shorts, my bib #, timing chip, body glide where needed, gel shots, sunglasses, hat or visor, and a light jacket. Everyone needs to arrive at the race at least an hour early.

The First Mile

Once I completed the first mile, I will be honest, I felt a bit nervous, but I was ready to apply all of my training for a safe and injury free race.

I found myself looking around and thinking, "Wow, the number of participants in this race is amazing." I started my race in the section with my pace group.

How to Pace yourself:

It's easy to feel invincible during the first couple of miles so here are a few tips to pace yourself during this part of the race.

- Don't exert all of your energy
- Maintain proper running form
- Focus on your pace

Find a way to internally motivate yourself with a scripture, music, quote, etc.

- Utilize your watch with special pace tracking feature
- You will know that you are running too hard if you are running beyond the pace you have trained for. For example, when I run too fast, I tire very easily, this affects my pace.

The first five miles felt a bit congested due to the number of runners, 44,000, to be exact. Despite feeling closed up, I felt very strong for the first five miles of the run, using the run/walk method.

Mile 9

By this time some of the people were spread out more in the race, I could better see my surroundings. While focusing on my pace, I looked to my left and observed a female runner, looking pretty focused while running. She never turned her head to the left nor the right, but at the same time, I noticed something trickling down her legs. Oh well, I guess she didn't get a chance to take that bathroom break earlier.

"Don't worry, keep running."

Mile 13: Halfway Through!

At this point, I was feeling like a real celebrity, making it to the halfway point of the marathon. Everywhere I turned there were many people. Babies, children, teens, and grandparents were lined up on each side of the race. Normally, the runners are coming through the center of the street. Someone was either holding up a big sign, or screaming something like,

"Good job, you go girl!" Or they would extend their hands to high-five me as I ran or walked by. There were even people shaking bells and playing drums. How exciting! I was feeling good about completing half of the race, but was also beginning to feel some rotating pain from one leg to the other. When I stopped at the next water station, I drank a cup of Gatorade and I stretched my legs a bit. Through the pain, I was focused on my goal time of five hours to complete the marathon and I continued to recite my favorite scripture, *"I can do all things through Christ which strengthens me."* Phil 4:13

Mile 21:

Ooh, wee! At this point in the Marathon I felt I had bitten off more than I could chew. It felt like my legs were in quick sand, and I was running but going nowhere. My lower body felt heavy, and all I wanted was some relief. At the moment I thought about giving up, I noticed a man with a prosthetic leg pass me. Suddenly, I remembered Matthew 24:13 that says, *"But he who endures to the end shall be saved."*

I fought really hard to stay focused because people all around me were having challenges in this race. Some were crying, or experiencing some form of injury, while others were being taken away in ambulances.

At one low point, I slowly reached into the back pocket of my shorts to take a gel shot, when a young lady from the crowd shouted, "Don't you stop now, you have come too far, you can do it!" I was too tired to explain what I was doing, so I just nodded my head in agreement with what she said. I appreciated her support. I found it strengthening so I prayed and stretched my legs and arms.

Suddenly, I remembered a song I like, "Ain't No Stopping Us Now" (McFadden & Whitehead). With renewed strength, I started back on my course of running and focused once again on maintaining my form and finishing the race within five hours. *"But they that wait upon the Lord shall renew their strength, they shall mount up with wings as eagles; they shall run, and not be weary; and they shall walk, and not faint."* Isaiah 40:31

The Finish Line!

Oh, Glory, I can see the finish sign. During the final stretch I pressed my way to the finish. I held my chin up, pumped my arms back and forth and ran as fast as I could with big strides. Once I crossed the finish line, I said, "Hallelujah! Thank you, Jesus, for helping me to finish that tough course." I did pass and survive the test of endurance. Someone greeted me with a large silver poncho, and a medal was placed around my neck. I was so grateful for the volunteer who assisted me in removing the timing chip from my shoe. My legs were so heavy from the run that it was too difficult for me to bend down that low to remove it myself. "Team work makes the dream work!"

Wow, I completed my first marathon with a time of 5:07:42 (5 hours 7 minutes and 42 seconds). My average speed per mile (also called pace per mile) was 11:44 (11 minutes and 44 seconds) in 2003.

Finishing this marathon was a victory for me. Following this awesome race, I decided that I wanted to take my method of running to another level!

I was ready for my next project. I heard some fellow runners talk about the popular, "Indianapolis Mini Marathon." I decided to register and run this race.

This half marathon was the most entertaining and scenic race in which I had ever participated in my running career. I completed my first half marathon in May of 2004 at the Indianapolis Life 500 Festival Mini Marathon.

CHAPTER EIGHT:

MY MARATHON RESUME

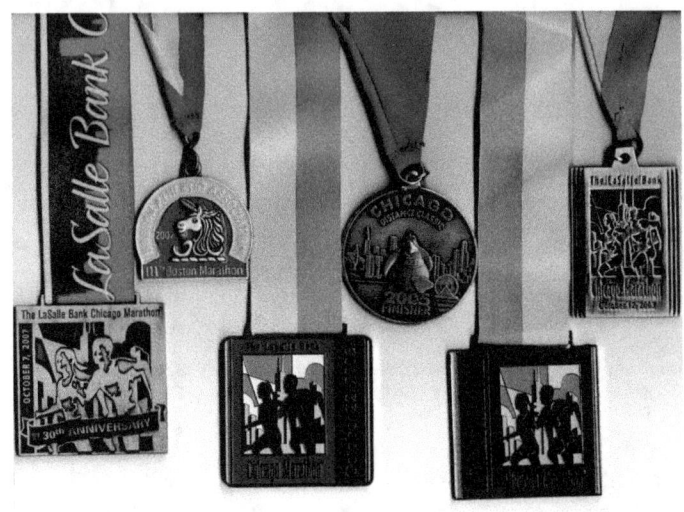

After the first marathon I was hooked! I also progressed from a run/walker to a runner. A runner doesn't stop for walking breaks as frequent as run/walkers. For instance: a run walker may run (when timer goes off on watch) for 10 minutes and walk for 2 minutes or run for 5 minutes and walk for 1 minute throughout the course of race. Here is a list of marathons that I completed over the next few years.

- Second- Chicago Marathon in Oct of 2004 with a completion time of 4:36:57 (4 hours, 36 minutes, and 57 seconds) and a Pace Per Mile time of 10:33 (10 minutes and 33 seconds).
- Third- Chicago Marathon in October of 2005 with a completion time of 4:44:53 and a Pace Per Mile time of 10:52
- Fourth- Chicago Marathon in October of 2006 with a completion time of 4:43:25 and a Pace Per Mile time of 10:49
- Fifth- Chicago Marathon in Oct of 2007 with a completion time of

5:19:36 and a Pace Per Mile time of 12:12

- Sixth- Boston Marathon in April of 2007 with a completion time of 4:40:32 and a Pace Per Mile time of 10:40

TO GOD BE THE GLORY!

References/Suggested Reading

The Holy Bible King James Version

The Holy Bible New King James Version

www.chicagoendurancesports.com

www.runnersworld.com/injury-prevention-recovery/benefits-of-massage-for-runners

Benefits of Massage for Runners by Susan Paul, Runner's World, © 2013

"6 Tips to Find the Perfect Pace"

By Fara Rosenzweig www.Active.com

Runner's World Magazine by Rodale Inc.

www.About.com "Running and Jogging: Best Foods for Runners", by Christine Luff, © 2013

ABOUT THE AUTHOR

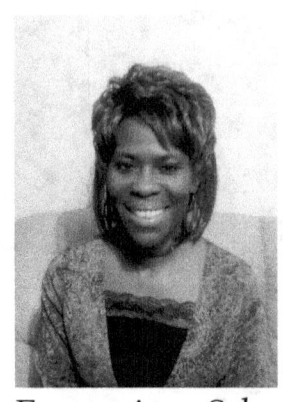

Yolanda is a dancer and choreographer. She was born in Chicago, Illinois where she received training in dance under the teaching of Rosalyn Acevedo of the Divine Expressions School of Dance in 2005; Renee Gray of the Praise Party School of Dance in 2007 and Jocelyn Richard of the Praise Dance Life in 2012. She has attended many conferences and workshops that teach choreography of dance. The classes included: ballet, modern dance, technique in dance, and flag worship. Yolanda's gifts and talents began to grow spiritually under the leadership of Eric Susberry, Pastor of Elim Christian Church. Yolanda has choreographed and danced for women's and church events, appreciations, dance concerts, conferences, workshops and outreach events as well. Yolanda is one of the founders and the leader of the J.O.Y.D. (Joyful Obedient Yielded Dancer) Dance Ministry in Chicago, Illinois. She is using her gift to spread the gospel through the use of movement. In 2008, she graduated and received her License as a Minister of Dance from the Eagles International Training Institute, under the leadership of Apostle Dr. Pamela Hardy.

In 2010, the Lord called Yolanda to reach the nations as a missionary in Trinidad and Africa. Yolanda is currently serving as the Director of the Dance Ministry at Elim Christian Church in Chicago.

Yolanda Hill

How I Ran My First Marathon

Yolanda Hill